Divided by Conflict, United by Compassion

The National Museum of Civil War Medicine

Terry Reimer

NMCWM Press

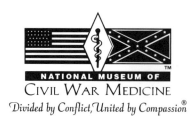

CIVIL WAR MEDICINE
Divided by Conflict, United by Compassion®

Published by: The NMCWM Press
                 The National Museum of Civil War Medicine, Inc.
                 P.O. Box 470
                 Frederick, MD 21705
                 Phone: 1-800-564-1864
                 Fax: 1-301-695-6823
                 www.civilwarmed.org
                 email: museum@civilwarmed.org

ISBN# 0-9712233-2-7

The NMCWM is a not-for-profit 501(c)(3) corporation

Book design by: Scott Edie, E Graphics

Photographers: Scott Edie, Larry Ketron, John Reimer, Terry Reimer, Ryan Rokicki, Laurence Sorcher, Karen Thomassen, Kari Turner

Printed by: Progressive Printing & Graphics, Martinsburg, West Virginia

Printed and bound in the United States of America

Funding for this book was provided by the G. Frank Thomas Foundation, Inc., Frederick, Maryland

First Edition

Cover photographs and design by Scott Edie, E Graphics

Foreword

Gordon E. Dammann, D.D.S.
Chairman, NMCWM Board of Directors

What began in 1971 as a hobby turned into a passion by 1988. My original idea was to collect and catalog medical artifacts from the Civil War. In doing so, the true story of medicine at that time would be told. During those first years of collecting I met many Civil War collectors at yearly shows. One gave me some very good advice: "You are not a collector of items. You are a caretaker of these items for a period of time." A caretaker sees that the items in his or her care are maintained for the education of future generations. This is why the idea for a museum came into being.

In every collection of Civil War artifacts there are one or two pieces that take on a special meaning for the owner. In my collection one such piece is an artificial leg that belonged to Civil War veteran Peleg Bradford of the 1st Maine Heavy Artillery. Along with the leg came twelve letters that he had written to his intended bride, Cynthia McPherson. It was during the siege of Petersburg that Peleg became a victim of the ravages of war. On June 17, 1864, he was wounded in the leg. Two surgical procedures were performed, one to amputate the limb and the second to combat the effects of hospital gangrene. In his last letter to Cynthia, Peleg explained that he had been wounded and "is not a whole man." He therefore would not expect her to be held by their betrothal.

After a long search, I was able to find out more about Peleg through contact with the Bradford family historian, Richard Bradford. Mr. Bradford was able to relate a first-hand account of Peleg's wounding: "Grandfather was crouched in one of those shallow rifle pits and a piece of gravel fell inside his right shoe. He was reaching inside the shoe with his index finger, trying to dislodge the particle with his right knee pulled up close to his head, and he always thought a Rebel sharpshooter aimed for his head and missed, but the Minié ball shattered his knee, and he said his leg started jumping around like a beheaded chicken. The first amputation became infected with gangrene and the next one was halfway up his thigh."

Peleg must have thought his life had come to an end. His body was disfigured and his family was far away. His intended bride was not there to give him the love he needed, assuring him that losing his leg did not change her feelings for him. I wonder how many times he lay in bed looking at the stump of a leg and cursing the situation. Somehow he managed to find the courage to pick up his life and begin again.

Peleg returned home to Maine, married Cynthia and started a family. Richard Bradford's last letter to me has the following quote: "He brought no single item of Army gear home with him and was, in fact, left with such an aversion to dealing with death that he never allowed a firearm of any kind in his house...Yes, I think he had a certain pride in having served. He was a G.A.R. member and was glad to reunite with his old comrades-in-arms. He recognized the men he fought against being like him and often said he'd like to meet the Johnny who shot him, not for revenge, but to have a chance to compare notes and get to know him as a man."

What began as an acquisition for my collection turned out to be an in-depth look at a veteran of the Civil War. I believe it is the responsibility of every collector to find out as much as possible about each item he acquires. In this way we keep alive the history of the gallant men, both Union and Confederate, who gave of themselves to make this the country we have today. Creating a museum was the next step in this worthwhile process.

On a sunny Saturday in October 2000, my impossible dream came true. The newly-renovated and expanded National Museum of Civil War Medicine opened its doors to the public. It was a proud day for all who had worked so hard to make this dream a reality. I can't begin to thank all who helped with this project, however, I want to thank my beloved family, Karen, Greg and Doug, for standing by me all these years. Without their love and support this impossible dream would not have come true.

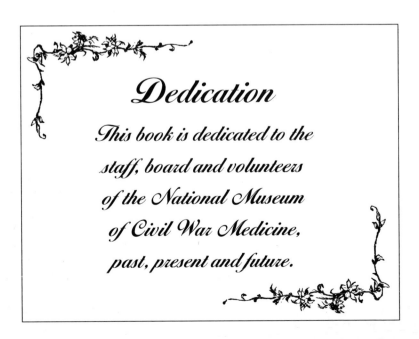

Dedication

This book is dedicated to the staff, board and volunteers of the National Museum of Civil War Medicine, past, present and future.

Contents

Introduction

The National Museum of Civil War Medicine is dedicated exclusively to the study and interpretation of the medical aspects of the Civil War. It is a story of care and healing, courage and devotion amidst the death and destruction of war. It is also a story of major advances that changed medicine forever and of the thousands of men and women who risked everything to make a terrible situation better. Through the dedication, innovation and devotion of Civil War surgeons and medical support staff on both sides of the conflict, the foundation for today's modern military medicine was laid. Their tenacity and compassion to heal stemmed a death rate that could have easily been twice the 620,000.

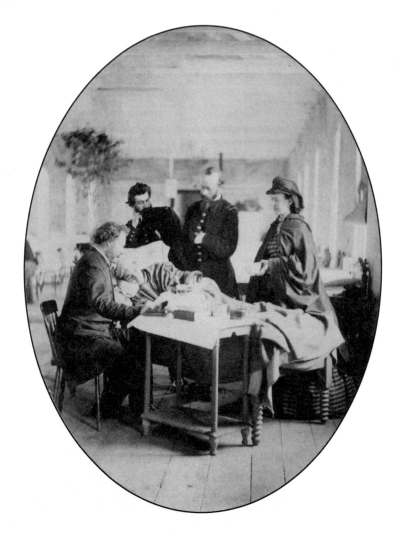

The Beginnings

The creation of The National Museum of Civil War Medicine started as the idea of Gordon E. Dammann, D.D.S., whose collection of medical artifacts from the Civil War forms the core of the Museum's holdings. Dr. Dammann began collecting in 1971, and felt that a museum would be a good way to share his collection and the story of Civil War medicine with the public. With the help of F. Terry Hambrecht, M.D.; Sam Kirkpatrick, M.D.; John Olson; the Reverend John Schildt; and Thomas Adrian Wheat, M.D., the idea began to take shape. The Museum was incorporated in 1990, and the board of directors began the search for a location for the Museum, selecting the area near Antietam National Battlefield in Washington County, Maryland. However, delays in reaching an agreement with the National Park Service led the board to widen its search for a permanent home for the nascent Museum.

With the support of the Governor of Maryland and the Mayor and Board of Aldermen of Frederick City, in August 1993 the board chose to locate the National Museum of Civil War Medicine in Frederick, Maryland. Placing the Museum in Frederick was a strategic decision designed to attract the large number of tourists who visit the area every year. The city is centrally located within a thirty-minute drive to five major Civil War battlefields: Gettysburg, Pennsylvania; Harpers Ferry, West Virginia; Antietam, Maryland; South Mountain, Maryland; and Monocacy, Maryland. It is also near the major tourist destinations of Washington, D.C., and Baltimore, Maryland. The Carty Building, a city-owned building in the heart of Frederick's historic district, was chosen as the site of the Museum.

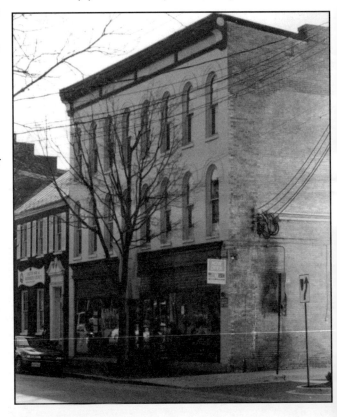

Once a location was established, the board began a fund-raising campaign and hired the Museum's first executive director, Burton K. Kummerow, in March 1994. Local banks, the City of Frederick, Frederick County and numerous private citizens donated to the cause. The board and staff's efforts received a major boost when the State

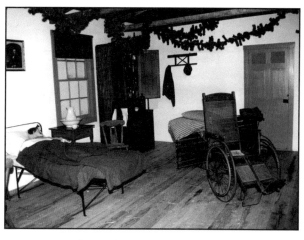

of Maryland awarded the Museum a $1 million challenge grant for the much-needed renovation of the historic Carty Building.

A membership program was instituted and the Museum began publishing its quarterly newsletter, *Surgeon's Call*. On June 15, 1996, the first exhibits were opened to the public, replacing the temporary displays that had been set up in the front windows of the building. The exhibits included dioramas, cases and informational panels on recruiting, camp life, medical evacuation, field hospitals, pavilion hospitals, and the home-front. The displays were highlighted by a Confederate ambulance on loan from the Lincoln Memorial University, a nine-teenth-century holding coffin, stretchers, amputation kits, uniforms of medical personnel, and numerous other medical and surgical items.

The National Museum of Civil War Medicine had difficulty raising the needed $1 million to match the State of Maryland's grant for the renovation of the building and was given an additional two years to complete the task. JaNeen M. Smith replaced Burton K. Kummerow as executive director in September 1996, and a new period of growth followed. Additional staff members were hired, new exhibits were added to the gallery, a website was launched, and public restrooms were built. The Museum also applied to participate in the Museum Assessment Program of the American Association of Museums.

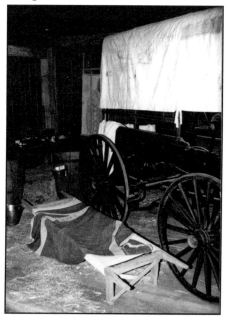

In July 1997, the Museum received a $1 million gift from the Judge Edward S. Delaplaine Charitable Trust, fully matching the State of Maryland's challenge grant. Plans for the renovation of the building and the design and installation of new exhibits began in earnest.

The Carty Building

The Museum building is located on lots 41 and 42 of the original plat of Frederick City, laid out in 1745. James Whitehill acquired the property in 1832 and occupied it until after the Civil War. He established a furniture and undertaking business on the site and operated a lumber yard and planing mill at the rear of the property. In the nineteenth century, it was common for furniture makers to also act as undertakers, since the main job of undertakers was to provide coffins and caskets. Whitehill's business flourished during the Civil War; he provided a large number of caskets and wooden burial markers to General Hospital #1, which was located at the Hessian Barracks in Frederick, Maryland. Dr. Richard Burr, Embalming Surgeon for the U.S. Army, used part of the property after the battles of South Mountain and Antietam in September 1862.

After the war, Whitehill sold the lumber yard and planing mill at the back of the property to John C. Hardt and Hiram Keefer, and the furniture and undertaking business to Clarence C. Carty. In 1892, Clarence Carty demolished the existing building at the front of the property and rebuilt a larger one on the site, which encompasses the western two-thirds of the present building. The rear section of the present building dates to the 1830's. In 1922, the store was renovated, expanding the existing building to the east and incorporating a small brick building that had stood on that site. The current facade of the Museum dates to 1922 and has eight arched widows on both the second and third floors, and a plate glass storefront on the first floor. The Carty family continued to operate a furniture and undertaking business on the site until 1978. The City of Frederick bought the property in 1989.

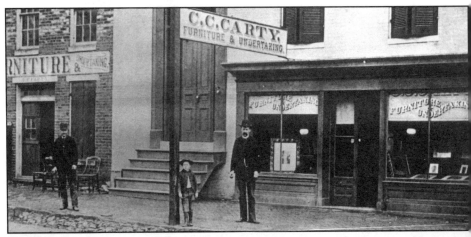

C. C. Carty's Furniture and Undertaking, c. 1884. Pictured, l-r, are Willie Keller, handyman, Henry E. Carty, Clarence C. Carty. Courtesy of Frances Randall.

Building Renovations & The Temporary Location

By early 1998, a team for the Museum renovation project was assembled. The board of directors chose the architectural firm of Martinez & Johnson and the general contractor Struever Brothers, Eccles & Rouse, Inc., to renovate the building. The exhibit design build firm of Kund & Associates was chosen to design, fabricate and install the state-of-the-art exhibits. Rounding out the team was Creative Display Installation, Inc., specializing in the construction of dioramas and environmental displays. Anatoliy Shapiro of Shapiro's Art Studio was chosen to paint the murals for the exhibits.

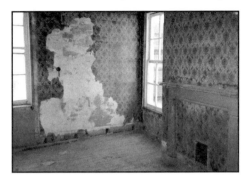

The historic Carty building on East Patrick Street was in need of major renovation and stabilization. Funding for the improvements came from the State of Maryland's $1 million challenge grant and the matching $1 million from the Judge Edward S. Delaplaine Charitable Trust. The older section in the rear of the structure needed to be rebuilt from the inside, and the front section was in need of structural stabilization and modernization for use as a Museum. The third floor of the structure had seen little use and had sustained considerable water damage. The entire roof needed to be replaced, and all of the utilities had to be upgraded with museum-quality equipment.

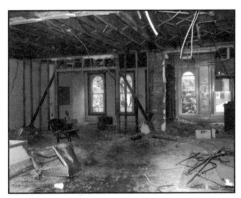

Renovations to the outside of the building were steered by the guidelines of the Frederick Historic District Commission and by a Maryland Historical Trust easement on the building. Little was to be changed on the exterior, other than the removal of a modern side stairway, second floor deck, and door. The historic windows and decorative trim were to be repaired and repainted, and the brick repointed.

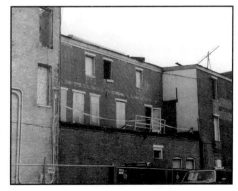

In order to facilitate the renovation, the Museum itself had to be relocated to a temporary site, since it was decided that the exhibits, store and research library should remain open to the public. A city-owned building on Adventist Drive in Frederick was chosen as the temporary Museum site, and exhibits were re-designed and installed at

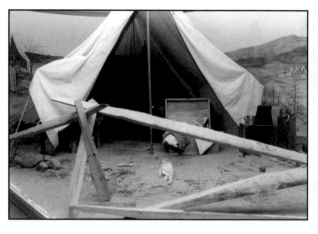

this location. In April 1999, the collections, Dispensary Store, research library and offices were moved to this facility, and the Museum was re-opened to the public within a week of the move.

During the renovation of the East Patrick Street building, preserving the historic nature of the structure was paramount. The exterior was restored in accordance with the Frederick Historic District Commission and the Maryland Historic Trust. In the interior, what remained of the historic floor plan was retained wherever possible, especially on the third floor. Ramps were designed to connect the differing floor levels between the 1830 and 1890 sections of the building. Existing nineteenth century interior shutters were restored for use in the Conference Room, and other historic building materials were re-used throughout the exhibits. An early passenger elevator was still in working order and was retained for staff use.

Also in April of 1999, the Museum received a $750,000 grant from the State of Maryland for the design and construction of the new exhibits in the renovated building. A team featuring the exhibit designers, board members and staff planned the layout and the content of the exhibits. The restrictions imposed by

the floor plan of the historic structure had to be considered in the design process, but the goal of the team was to tell the story of Civil War medicine in

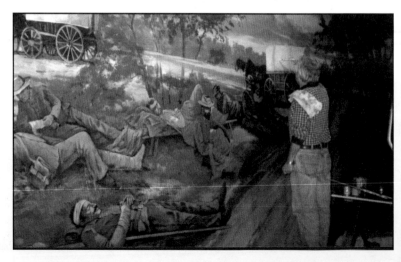

much the same order as it would have been experienced by the soldiers themselves. In the finalized layout, the first gallery establishes the context for the Museum by discussing the state of medicine and medical education at the beginning of the war. The remaining galleries follow the soldiers through recruitment, camp life, the evacuation of the wounded, field dressing stations, field hospitals, and pavilion hospitals. The last gallery highlights specific subjects such as indigenous plants used by the surgeons, dentistry, Naval medicine, and the Civil War hospitals in Frederick, while allowing room for future exhibits.

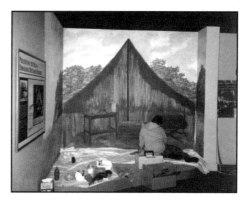

On October 21, 2000, the newly-renovated Museum opened its doors to the public. In addition to the two floors of exhibit galleries, the Museum features an expanded Dispensary Store at the front of the building; the Delaplaine Randall Conference Room on the second floor; a secure, climate-controlled collections room, a research center and administrative offices on the third floor. Since the re-opening, additional exhibits have been added that study the embalming of the dead, apothecary wagons, and nursing during the Civil War. At present, plans are progressing for an expanded exhibit on the hospitals in Frederick and a comparative look at modern military medicine.

On November 15, 2002, executive director JaNeen Smith retired and was succeeded by George Wunderlich, the Museum's director of education. Ms. Smith had been instrumental in implementing the renovation, hiring additional staff for the expanded Museum, and acquiring full accreditation from the American Association of Museums, helping to ensure the success of the young institution. Mr. Wunderlich has an extensive background in history and brings a boundless enthusiasm to the position, characteristics that will enable the Museum to continue to grow and expand in the future.

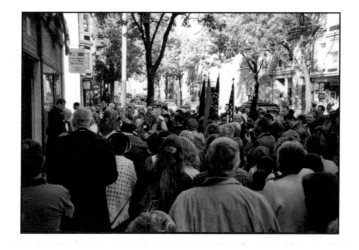

AAM Accreditation

In November 2002, the Museum was awarded the highest honor a museum can receive: full accreditation by the American Association of Museums (AAM). Accreditation certifies that a museum operates according to standards set forth by the museum profession, manages its collections responsibly and provides quality service to the public. Less than five percent of the nation's museums have been awarded AAM accreditation. The National Museum of Civil War Medicine is one of the youngest museums in the nation to have been granted full accreditation.

Accreditation is one of several programs offered by the American Association of Museums to help museums achieve and maintain current standards of quality and excellence in the profession. AAM is a national organization, with its headquarters in Washington, D.C., that has served the museum profession since 1906.

National Museum of Civil War Medicine's AAM Accreditation Timeline

Early 1997:   CAP (Conservation Assessment Program), general conservation surveys of the Museum's collection and the building.

Late 1997:   MAP I (Museum Assessment Program, Institutional Assessment), review of the Museum's management and operations.

Fall 1999:   MAP III (Museum Assessment Program, Public Dimension Assessment), review of the Museum's public perception and involvement.

August 2000:   Museum enters AAM Accreditation Program.

January 2001:   MAP Governance Assessment (Museum Assessment Program, Pilot Project), review of the governing authority of a museum, examining its roles and responsibilities to evaluate how well it is functioning.

November 2001:   Interim AAM accreditation awarded to the Museum

November 2002:   Full AAM accreditation granted to the Museum.

The Building's Elevators

The oldest elevator in the Carty building is an open freight elevator located in the northwest corner of the 1830's portion of the structure. It was installed between 1892 and 1897. A metal plate on the elevator notes that it was manufactured by James Bates of No. 1 President Street in Baltimore, Maryland, and was patented in 1871, with a reissue of the patent in 1876. Most of the parts have survived, including the elevator itself, its wooden mortise and tenon support structure, wooden cog and pulley wheels and hemp rope. The freight elevator is no longer in operation but is preserved in place and is located within the collections room on the third floor of the Museum.

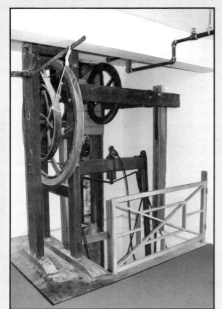

The original passenger elevator in the building is located in the southeast corner of the 1922 portion of the

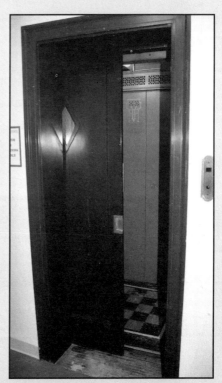

structure. It was installed between 1929 and 1934 and retains most of its original features, including the mechanism, flooring and decorative paint. It is still in working order and is used by the Museum staff.

Exhibits

The National Museum of Civil War Medicine has over 7,000 square feet of exhibit space spread over two floors, featuring immersion exhibits that bring the visitor into the setting and vividly illustrate different aspects of Civil War medicine by minimizing the physical barriers that usually separate the visitor from the exhibit. The galleries examine key concepts of medicine during the war, including the medical education of the surgeons, the recruitment and everyday life of the soldiers, evacuation of the wounded, battlefield medicine and hospital care, dentistry, pharmaceuticals, embalming, and Naval medicine. The exhibits combine large graphic panels, full-scale dioramas, murals, sound effects, reproduction items, original artifacts housed in custom-made cases, and hands-on displays to tell the story of Civil War medicine.

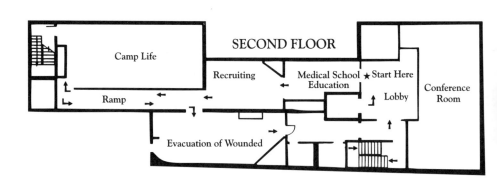

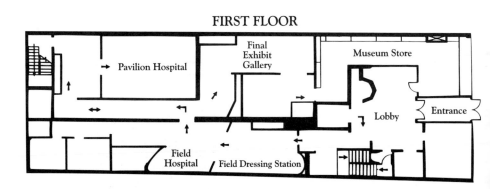

Peleg Bradford

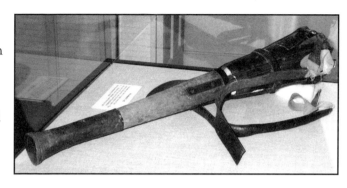

I n the course of planning the exhibits the design team chose to high-light the words and experiences of one soldier, Peleg Bradford of the 1st Maine Heavy Artillery, and use them to navigate visitors through the Museum. From his illness in camp to being wounded in battle to his recovery in the hospital system, Peleg's experiences perfectly illustrate the medical care most soldiers received. Using Peleg's own descriptions helps add a humanizing touch to the exhibits. The quotes used in the panels come from letters that he wrote to Cynthia, his fiancée, that were preserved by his family in Maine.

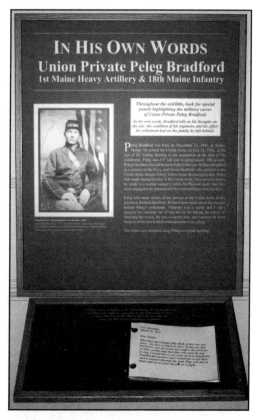

Peleg was wounded in the right knee during the siege of Petersburg, Virginia, in June 1864. As a result, his leg was amputated at mid-thigh and he spent months recuperating in the Columbian College Hospital in Washington, D.C. Once he recovered, he returned home to Maine, married Cynthia, and raised eight children. He worked as a shoemaker and also founded a successful sawmill. He died in 1919. Bradford's prosthetic leg is on display in the final gallery of the Museum.

Medical School Education Gallery

As the Civil War began, the practice of medicine was emerging from the "heroic era," with its theory of bringing a balance to the humors of the body. To that end, bleeding, cupping and purging were still practiced but were on the wane. Medical practitioners had no knowledge of germ theory or antiseptic practices, since both discoveries were still years away. Over forty medical schools existed in the United States before the war, and apprenticeships with established physicians were also common. The usual course of study in a medical school consisted of two terms of six-month lectures, with the second term often being a repeat of the first.

Featured items in this gallery include a bloodletting fleam, thermometer, microscope, stethoscope, medical school diplomas and lecture tickets, anatomical teaching specimens, and textbooks.

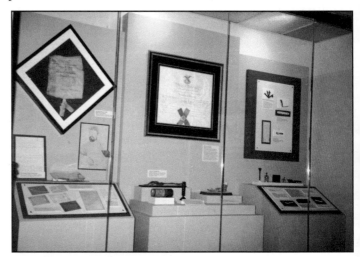

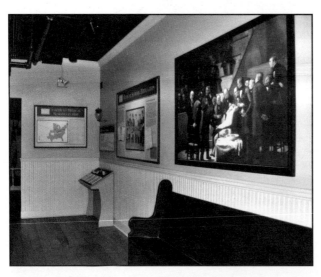

Surgeons

At the beginning of the Civil War, the Medical Corps of the United States Army consisted of one Surgeon General, thirty surgeons, and eighty-three assistant surgeons. Of these, twenty-four resigned their commissions to serve the Confederacy. By the end of the war, thousands of men served as surgeons or assistant surgeons on both sides of the struggle. All physicians were officers in their respective armies, surgeons being the equivalent of a major and assistant surgeons a captain or first lieutenant.

Over 12,000 physicians served the Union in some capacity, either in regiments, on ships, or as surgeons in the many hospitals. Approximately 6,500 of these were appointed as officers, and another 5,500 served as civilians under contract with the army. Contract surgeons, also called Acting Assistant Surgeons, were doctors in private practice, often men too infirm to go into the field, who signed on to help in hospitals on a contract basis.

An estimated 8,000 physicians served for the Confederacy; of these, approximately 6,800 were appointed, while at least 1,200 served on a contract basis.

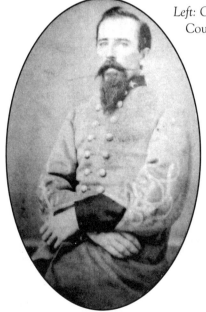

Left: Confederate Brigade Surgeon John Hays.
Courtesy of Jonathan O'Neal, M.D.

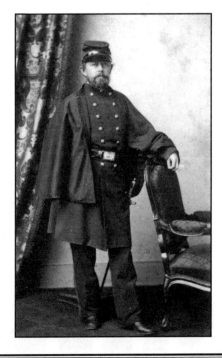

Right: Union Brigade Surgeon Reed B. Bontecue.
Courtesy of Gordon E. Dammann, D.D.S.

Recruiting & Enlisting Gallery

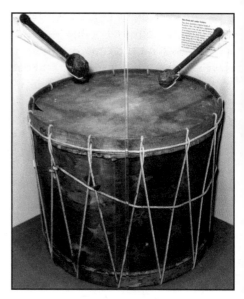

Army regulations required that all new recruits receive a thorough physical exam at the time of their enlistment. Occasionally the exam was very superficial, allowing recruits to enter the army with chronic diseases and physical defects that would affect their performance as a soldier. While some examining surgeons were conscientious, others were less so, allowing unsuitable men, and a number of women, into the armies. As the war progressed and the number of men willing to enlist dwindled, both the North and South resorted to instituting a draft to secure the large number of soldiers needed for the war.

Featured items in this gallery include a recruiting drum and broadsides, medical examination forms and regulation books, and photographs of surgeons.

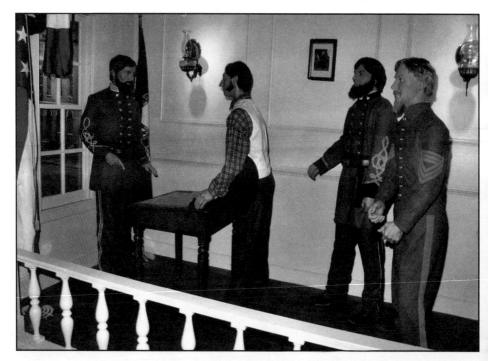

Smallpox

Smallpox was one of the many diseases challenging medical personnel during the Civil War. Unlike most other diseases, the surgeons of the time had an effective way to prevent smallpox using vaccination. They also controlled outbreaks through the isolation of its victims.

Inoculation for smallpox had been in widespread use since the 1720's, and vaccination was developed in 1798 by Edward Jenner. The cowpox serum was used because cowpox is a closely related disease and created a resistence to smallpox. Like inoculation, the vaccine was administered through a series of small cuts in the skin, usually in the arm.

Quarantine, vaccination, and the destruction of infected clothes and bedding were the primary tools used to control the spread of smallpox. Most hospitals had a separate ward, or even a separate hospital, in which to isolate the patients since the disease was known to be contagious.

Both Union and Confederate regulations required the vaccination of all troops. Since there had been no systemic vaccination of the civilian populations, many of the recruits had never been vaccinated or exposed to smallpox. Re-vaccination was recommended after seven years had elapsed from the last vaccination, or when men were directly exposed to the disease.

The best and purest source for vaccine was derived from the crust of cowpox pustules on cows or calves. The pressing demands of war often led authorities to institute programs that obtained the scabs from vaccinated humans. The Union medical dispensaries of the northern cities supplied vaccine virus in the form of crusts taken from vaccinated infants, each with a certificate listing the dispensary and the child's name.

In the Confederacy, many programs were set up to assure an adequate supply of vaccine scabs for the army. Every hospital had a medical officer whose job was to search the surrounding populace for children on whom they could propagate the virus. In at least one instance a small group of African American children were kept vaccinated to provide usable material. The children were vaccinated in six places in each arm. In two weeks the crusts were removed, wrapped in tin foil, and shipped to army surgeons.

Children and cows were the safest sources for crusts, but there were many documented instances where other methods were used. Surgeons often used the scabs from recently-vaccinated men to vaccinate other soldiers. Soldiers did the same among themselves, sharing the crusts and using knives to make the incisions in their arms. Some men even sent scabs home for the use of their families.

The preventive measures of vaccination and isolation taken by the Union and Confederate Medical Departments curbed the occurrence of smallpox during the war and averted any major outbreaks. The success of the vaccination of soldiers during the Civil War led to widespread vaccination of the civilian population after the war, further helping to control this serious disease.

Camp Life Gallery

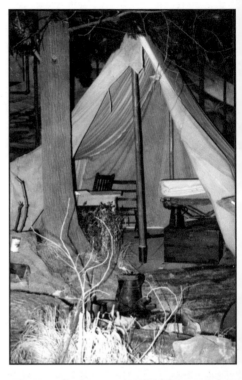

New recruits were sent to large camps to train to become soldiers. The first enemy they faced was disease. Healthy recruits became victims of illnesses that were easily spread due to the large number of people in the camps, the often unsanitary conditions, and the poor diet of the soldiers. Childhood diseases such as measles could devastate regiments, and many men succumbed to diarrhea and dysentery. Of the nearly 620,000 soldiers who died during the Civil War, two-thirds died not of bullets and bayonets, but of disease.

Featured items in this gallery include uniforms and personal items of medical officers and soldiers, games and diversions of camp, and the only known surviving surgeon's tent from the Civil War, which belonged to Surgeon John Wiley of the 6th New Jersey.

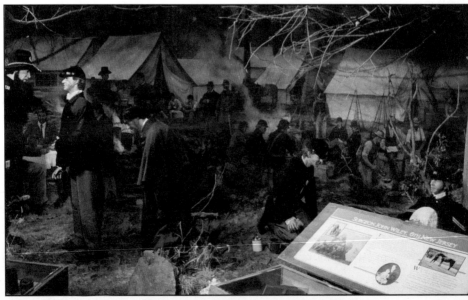

Diseases

Camp Fever: This term was used for all of the continuing fevers experienced by the army: typhoid fever, malarial remittent fever, and typho-malarial fever. The last named is a combination of elements from the first two diseases. This combination was considered the characteristic "camp fever" during the Civil War. Symptoms included a pronounced chill followed by an intermittent fever, abdominal tenderness and nausea, general debility, diarrhea, retention of urine, and furring of the tongue. If not checked, the disease could progress to emaciation, delirium, and prostration.

Diarrhea and Dysentery: Diarrhea was considered a specific disease during the Civil War, not a symptom of various diseases. Diarrhea and dysentery (diarrhea with bloody stools) were often combined during the war for record keeping purposes. They were by far the most common complaint of Civil War soldiers and also caused the most deaths and debility. Diarrhea was categorized as being either acute or chronic. Acute diarrhea was more dangerous, but the lingering affects of chronic diarrhea could remain with a person for the rest of his life. The causes, of which there were many, included poor rations, unsanitary conditions, food poisoning, bacteria, and a host of other diseases like scurvy.

Erysipelas: An acute inflammation of the skin and subcutaneous tissue caused by the bacterium *Streptococcus pyogenes.* It is characterized by reddening and severe inflammation and can lead to the formation of pustules. Erysipelas is usually accompanied by severe constitutional symptoms. It was often a complication from a wound or surgery.

Rheumatism: Rheumatism was also common both during and after the war. Again, there were two types–acute and chronic. Acute rheumatism is rheumatic fever and could be deadly. Chronic rheumatism was either a prolonged rheumatic fever or some type of reactive or rheumatoid arthritis.

Scurvy/Scorbutus: Scorbutus is another term for scurvy. Scurvy was a common condition afflicting Civil War soldiers. It is caused by a deficiency in vitamin C and is characterized by weakness, debility, anemia, spongy gums and edema. Fresh vegetables were the best preventative for scurvy, with potatoes and onions topping the list of vegetables preferred by the armies.

Typhoid Fever: Typhoid fever is spread by ingesting food or water contaminated with the bacterium *Salmonella typhi.* It is characterized by fever, severe debility, red skin lesions, intestinal disturbances, and delirium. Complications can include perforation of the intestines and pneumonia.

Medical Evacuation Gallery

At the beginning of the Civil War, neither army had established a system to transport wounded soldiers from the front lines to the field hospitals in the rear. In August of 1862, Jonathan Letterman, the Medical Director of the Army of the Potomac, created a highly-organized system of ambulances and trained stretcher bearers designed to evacuate the wounded as quickly as possible. A similar plan was adopted by the Confederate Army. The Letterman plan remains the basis for present military evacuation systems.

Horses and mules were essential to the army and to the Medical Department, and veterinary medicine played an important role in the war. Large infirmaries were developed to treat animals too sick or worn down to be of immediate use. An estimated 1 million horses and mules died in service to the armies.

Featured items in this gallery include various stretchers for transporting the wounded, ambulance corps items, medicinal supply boxes and cabinets, the frock coat and boots belonging to Surgeon Louis Radzinsky of the 54th Massachusetts, and items related to the care of animals, including a veterinary surgical kit and bloodletting fleam.

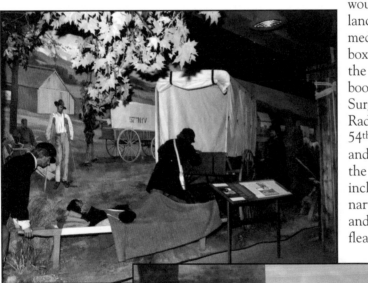

Surgeon Louis Radzinsky

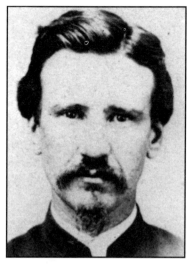

Union Surgeon Louis Daniel Radzinsky served with the 36th New York Infantry as a Surgeon's Mate from July to December 1861, then as a civilian contract surgeon from February 1862 until August 1864. He served in The U.S. General Hospital in Chester, Pennsylvania; the Broad and Cherry Streets Hospital in Philadelphia, Pennsylvania; and at the hospitals in Hilton Head and Morris Island, South Carolina.

On August 16, 1864, Radzinsky re-enlisted with the Army, joining the 54th Massachusetts Infantry. The 54th Massachusetts is the famous African American regiment featured in the film *Glory*. Radzinsky served as Assistant Surgeon with this regiment at Morris Island, Hilton Head, and Charleston, South

Union Surgeon Louis Daniel Radzinsky. Courtesy of Gordon E. Dammann, D.D.S.

Carolina. He was promoted to Surgeon on June 14, 1865 and transferred to the 104th United States Colored Troops, serving in Hilton Head and Beaufort, South Carolina. He resigned on February 5, 1866, and served again as a contract surgeon. Radzinsky later opened a private medical practice in McKeesport, Pennsylvania, and died on July 1, 1892.

The 54th Massachusetts Infantry

The 54th Massachusetts Infantry was organized in March 1863. It was primarily composed of free men and was one of the first African American units raised in the northern states. The principle battles in which this regiment participated were Olustee, Florida; James Island, Honey Hill, and Boykin's Mill, South Carolina; and at Fort Wagner, South Carolina, where they sustained a casualty rate of 25 percent. During the course of the war, over 179,000 African Americans served in the Union Army, with over 40,000 casualties.

Field Dressing Station Gallery

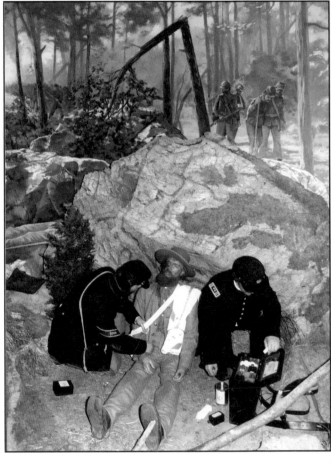

The first level of care received by a wounded soldier was at a field dressing station, located close to the fighting. Medical personnel bandaged wounds and administered whiskey for shock and morphine for pain. If the soldier was unable to return to battle, he was transported to a field hospital via ambulance or stretcher. The display depicts Union medical personnel attending to a wounded Confederate soldier. The location is modeled after the field dressing station of the 32nd Massachusetts Infantry near the Wheat Field at Gettysburg, Pennsylvania. It was common for medical personnel from both the North and South to treat the wounded from the other side. As Jonathan Letterman, Medical Director of the Army of the Potomac, said: "humanity teaches us that a wounded and prostrate foe is not then our enemy."

Featured items in this gallery include field medical cases, knapsacks and a

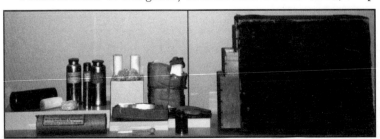

hospital backpack that were used by medical personnel at field dressing stations.

Monument

In the summer of 1996, the Museum adopted a monument on the Gettysburg National Military Park, through a program run by the National Park Service. Twice a year, Museum volunteers clear brush and perform a general cleanup of the site. The chosen monument commemorates the 32nd Massachusetts Volunteer Infantry field dressing station. It is located near the Wheat Field and is the only monument to a field dressing station on the Gettysburg National Military Park.

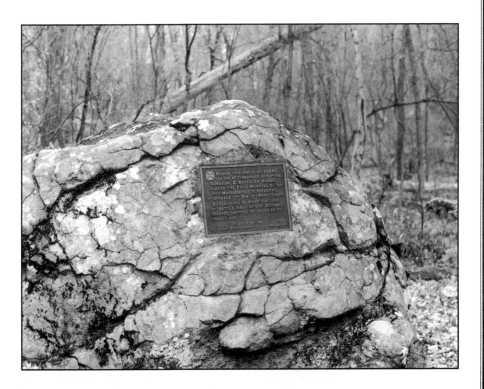

Field Hospital Gallery

At a field hospital, usually located in a barn or tent to the rear of the fighting, wounded soldiers were triaged into three categories: mortally wounded, slightly wounded, and surgical cases. Most surgeries were amputations and took place at the field hospitals. Of all the operations performed during the Civil War, 95 percent were done with the patient under some form of anesthesia, usually chloroform or ether. The large number of amputations performed during the war were the result of the severe nature of the wounds caused by the Minié ball, the number of wounded

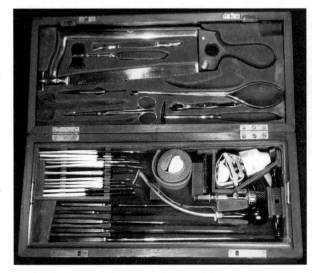

needing immediate treatment, and the often poor condition of the patients.

Featured items in this gallery include an amputation kit, a field pharmaceutical kit that belonged to Confederate Surgeon John Thomas Parker, various splints, tourniquets and medicine bottles, and a table used for performing surgeries during the Battle of Cedar Creek, Virginia.

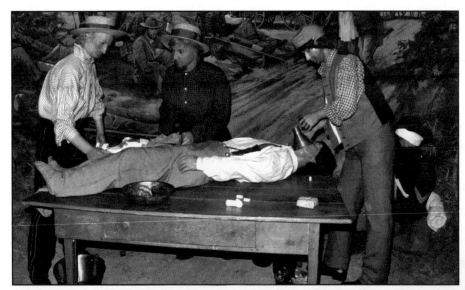

Anesthesia

Unfortunately, when most people think of Civil War surgery they envision a wounded soldier being forcibly held down while his arm or leg is amputated without the benefit of anesthesia. This Hollywood concept of Civil War surgery is far from accurate.

Sulfuric ether had been discovered in Europe in the 1830's. On October 16, 1846, William Thomas Green Morton, a dentist, exhibited the anesthetic properties of ether. With Morton holding the glass apparatus used to administer the ether, surgeon John Collins Warren removed a small tumor from the jaw of a patient. A public announcement was made on November 18, 1846, and ether was widely used within a few months. Chloroform, another anesthetic that had been discovered in 1832, was in common use soon after.

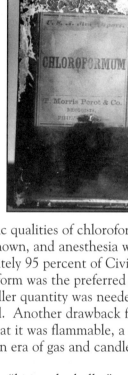

By the Civil War, the anesthetic qualities of chloroform and ether were well known, and anesthesia was used in approximately 95 percent of Civil War surgeries. Chloroform was the preferred anesthetic since a smaller quantity was needed and its effect was rapid. Another drawback for using ether was that it was flammable, a dangerous matter in an era of gas and candle lighting.

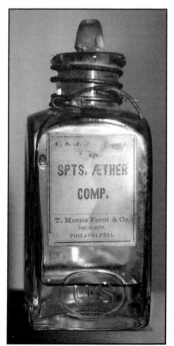

The myth about "biting the bullet" may have come from the fact that only a low dose of anesthetic was used during the Civil War, just enough to make the patient insensitive to pain. Surgeons worked quickly and could complete a major operation in a matter of minutes. Many men moaned and moved about due to the agitating effects of a light dose of anesthetic and some had to be held down by assistants, but they were unconscious and could not feel pain.

Amputation

The principal surgical procedure performed during the Civil War was amputation, mainly due to the extensive bone and tissue damage caused by the Minié ball. When estimates from both the Confederate and Union sides are combined, about 50,000 amputations were performed throughout the war. Most wounds were gunshot wounds, both from conical and round bullets, while the rest were from grapeshot, canister or other exploding shells wounds. Few men were treated for saber or bayonet wounds and even fewer for cannon ball wounds.

For most of the projectile injuries, the exit wound was often much larger than the entrance wound. The conical ball, or Minié ball, could inflict considerable damage to both bone and soft tissue due to its tendency to spin away from its long axis. Ricocheting or flattened bullets could create extensive lacerations and even carry foreign material into the wound.

The most common amputation sites on the body were the hand, thigh, lower leg, and upper arm. The likelihood of surviving an amputation depended on the distance of the operation site from the trunk of the body, and how long after the injury the surgery was performed. Generally, mortality rates dropped as the distance from the trunk of the body increased. For example, amputations at the wrist joint had a 10.4 percent death rate, while amputations at the shoulder joint had a 29.1 percent death rate.

Amputations were classified into three categories based on how soon after the injury the procedure was performed: primary, intermediary, and secondary. Primary amputations were done within forty-eight hours of the injury, intermediary amputations took place between three and thirty days after the wounding, and secondary amputations were performed more than thirty days after the injury. Intermediary amputations were the most dangerous because they were often done when the inflammation of the wound was at its greatest and the patient was suffering from its effects.

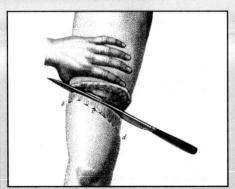

Circular amputation.   *Flap amputation.*
From The Illustrated Manual of Operative Surgery and Surgical Anatomy.

Pavilion Hospital Gallery

rior to the Civil War, any organized system of hospitalization was virtually unknown in the United States. With the large number of wounded and sick needing long-term care, a network of general hospitals was created in cities in both the North and the South. At first, large existing buildings were taken over for hospitals, but soon both armies constructed large pavilion-style hospitals that were clean, well ventilated, and highly efficient. Surgeons, hospital stewards, male nurses, female nurses, matrons, cooks, laundresses, and volunteers from civilian associations all contributed to the care of the sick and wounded. The quality of care that the patients received improved dramatically after the opening months of the war, and the general hospitals had an average mortality rate of 8 percent.

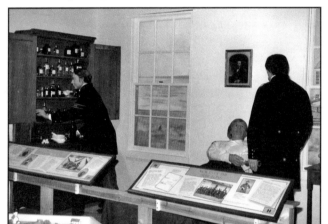

Featured items in this gallery include a large hospital drug chest, a Union garrison hospital flag, a scale model of the Hammond Hospital in Point Lookout, Maryland, crutches and prosthetic limbs, and items related to nursing during the war.

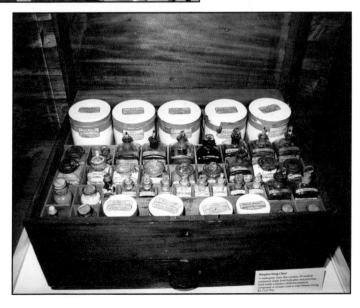

Hospital Gangrene

D uring the Civil War, the term "gangrene" was mainly used to refer to hospital gangrene. Hospital gangrene was very different from dry gangrene, which is the equivalent of modern-day gangrene and is caused by the disruption of circulation to a wound. Hospital gangrene was a contagious infection and was likely caused by a strain of the *Streptococcus* bacterium. It began as a discoloration near a wound that rapidly led to the progressive death of the surrounding tissue and was accompanied by a foul odor.

Cleanliness and good ventilation were seen as the best preventive measures for hospital gangrene, as crowded conditions were known to contribute to the outbreak and spread of the disease. Infected patients were removed from the wards, no dressings were reused, and each patient was given a new sponge which would often be cleaned. These procedures illustrate the surgeon's knowledge of the contagious nature of hospital gangrene and the beginnings of antiseptic practices, although the true mechanisms of antisepsis were unknown.

The treatments of hospital gangrene included cleaning the wound and removing all dead and infected tissue, then treating the surface with nitric acid, acid nitrate of mercury, or bromine. All these substances helped to kill the bacteria causing the infection, although the doctors did not understand why the treatments worked. Since applying these substances to a wound caused severe pain to the patient, chloroform was usually used as a general anesthetic before the treatment. The wound would be dressed with bandages after treatment. Hospital gangrene usually appeared after an amputation, especially in the lower extremities. The mortality rate from hospital gangrene was about 45 percent.

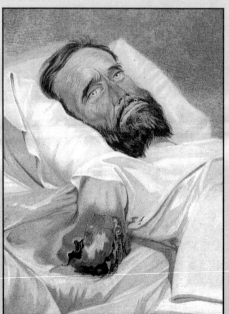

Hospital gangrene. From The Medical and Surgical History of the Civil War, Volume X.

Female Nurses

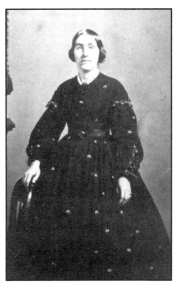

Women served as paid and volunteer nurses during the Civil War, and many others contributed their service through civilian organizations. Prior to the war, there were no formal training schools for nurses, male or female. Most medical care was focused in the home, and in this setting many women served as health care providers for their families. With the outbreak of war, women on both sides sought ways to put their valuable talents to work.

In the north, Dr. Elizabeth Blackwell organized a training program for female nurses in the city hospitals of New York. Dorothea Dix, a well-known mental health reformer, convinced the Army Medical Bureau to establish a corps of female nurses with herself as its superintendent. Over the next four years, thousands of women served in the general hospitals, the field hospitals and on the hospital transport ships. Other women volunteered to serve with the U. S. Sanitary Commission and the U. S. Christian Commission.

Mrs. Marsh, matron at the Judiciary Square Hospital, Washington, D.C. Courtesy of Gordon E. Dammann, D.D.S.

In the south, no formal training programs for nurses were established. Some women, like Ella Newsom, volunteered in city hospitals before offering their services to the army. In September 1862 the Confederate Congress, recognizing the contributions of these women, passed an Act authorizing the enlistment of female hospital workers. This Act classified the positions as chief, assistant and ward matrons with the monthly salaries of forty, thirty-five, and thirty dollars respectively.

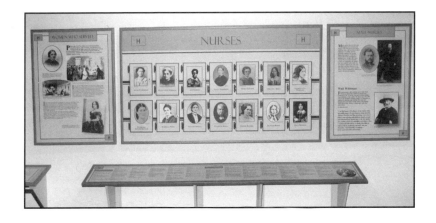

The Sister Nurses

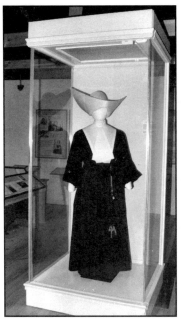

At the outbreak of the Civil War, communities of religious women were the only well-established groups which could transmit a heritage of knowledge, skills and management within an organized system of nursing. At least twenty-one different communities from twelve separate Catholic orders contributed the services of over six hundred sister nurses during the war. These sisters served hospitals, battlefields, camps and prisons for the armies of both the Union and the Confederacy.

Male Nurses

Many nurses who served in the hospitals were convalescent soldiers who were given extra duties until they were able to return to their regiment. If a soldier showed particular aptitude for nursing duties, the surgeons would often request that he be reassigned to hospital work. In 1863, the Union Veteran Reserve Corps (Invalid Corps) was established for soldiers who were unfit for active duty due to wounds or disease, but who were still able to perform limited service. The Veteran Reserve Corps supplied nurses, clerks, ward masters, guards and cooks to the general hospitals.

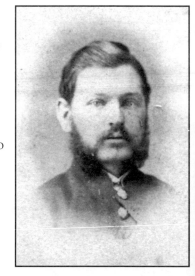

L. A. Thorpe, head nurse at Foster Hospital, New Bern, North Carolina. Courtesy of Gordon E. Dammann, D.D.S.

Hospital Trains

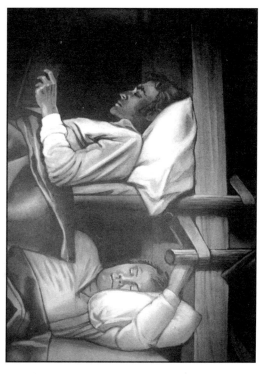

Many wounded soldiers were transported by rail to the pavilion hospitals established in larger urban areas. As early as August of 1861, railroad cars were being modified to transport the wounded; the first such cars were developed after the battle of Wilson's Creek, Missouri. By 1863, cars specifically produced for medical transportation were being built by the Philadelphia Railroad Company. While there was no standard design used for these cars, most followed the same general pattern. Patients were placed on stretchers in long rows inside the cars. The stretchers were suspended by vulcanized rubber rings which helped provide additional comfort for the patients by absorbing shock and creating a smoother ride.

The layout of the Museum's exhibit galleries was complicated by the fact that the floor levels do not line up between the different sections of the historic building. Two large ramps were incorporated into the structure and into the interpretation as well. The ramp on the first floor is designed to look like a typical hospital railroad car. Both walls have murals depicting a wide array of patients being transported to a hospital. Informational panels and sound effects complete the display.

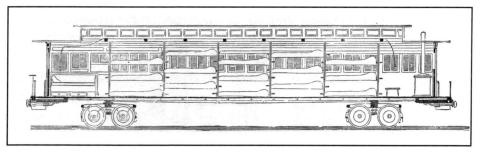

Hospital train car. From The Medical and Surgical History of the Civil War, Volume XII.

Final Exhibit Gallery

T he last exhibit area depicts a variety of subjects relating to Civil War medicine, including dental care during the Civil War, Naval medicine, an apothecary wagon, herbal medicines, the issues of death and embalming, the hospitals in Frederick after the battle of Antietam, and a look at military medicine in the past, present and future.

Featured items in this gallery include dental instruments, a mortar and pestle from the Navy hospital ship *Red Rover* and other items from Naval medical personnel, an embalming kit, a Civil War-era holding coffin, and a replica of an 1864 Autenrieth medicine wagon.

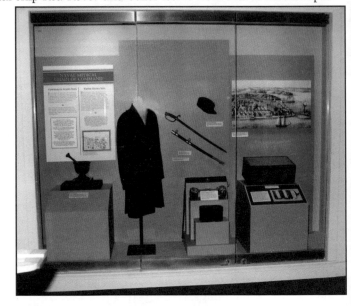

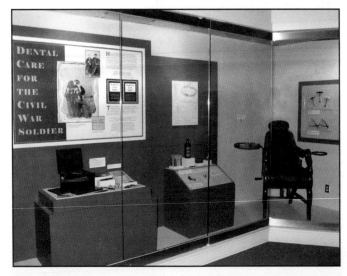

Autenrieth Medicine Wagon

Shortly after the war began, medical personnel of both the Union and Confederate armies recognized the difficulties of supplying their vast armies with proper medicines and medical supplies. Packing medical supplies into large chests or trunks and transporting them in wagons of the supply train often rendered items inaccessible when they were needed most. Additionally, transporting medical supplies in Army supply wagons proved wasteful as many of the bottles containing medicines were broken or damaged during transport.

An early medicine wagon was constructed in 1862 according to the plans and instructions of Union Medical Director Jonathan Letterman. In 1864, the Union Medical Board approved the Autenrieth wagon for field use. The top-heavy nature of the wagon caused some early problems, but once its design was perfected, it met with widespread approval. The Autenrieth wagon was unique in that it contained sliding shelves and drawers to hold medicines and supplies as well as a sliding flat work surface that could be pulled out when the back of the wagon was opened. When the Civil War ended, the Union Medical Department considered this improved medical wagon to be one of its greatest accomplishments.

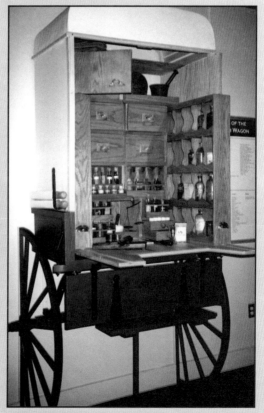

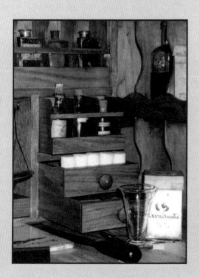

Embalming Surgeons

The process of embalming dates back to ancient Egypt, but it had not been widely used in the United States prior to the Civil War. It came into use during the war as a way to preserve bodies for shipment home. Due to the chemical injection method used in Civil War-era embalming, many embalmers were surgeons or pharmacists with a knowledge of chemical compounds. They often followed the armies, setting up their makeshift embalming stations near battlefields, hospitals and railroad stations.

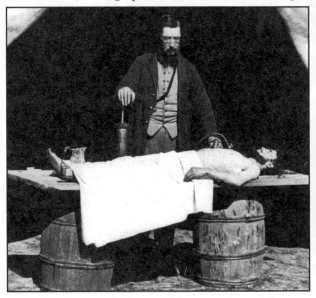

The most common procedure during the war was arterial embalming, where a pump was used to inject embalming fluid into either the carotid or femoral artery, attempting to get complete coverage throughout the body. Draining the blood was not necessary but was done on occasion. Many different chemicals were used for embalming fluid. Arsenic, bichloride of mercury, zinc chloride,

Dr. Richard Burr embalming a soldier. Courtesy of the Library of Congress.

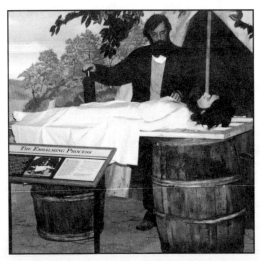

creosote, turpentine, and nitrate of potassium are some examples. Red dye was added to the mixture to give the body a more natural coloration.

It is estimated that between 10,000 and 40,000 soldiers were embalmed during the war. As a result, the procedure became more accepted and more common after the war. Undertakers gradually took over the task, ending the short era of the embalming surgeons.

Coffins and Transportation

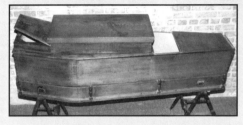

During the Civil War, the Federal and Confederate governments did not take responsibility for having soldiers' bodies shipped home for burial. Interment took place as soon as possible, in shallow graves with temporary markers. Families could arrange to have the bodies of their loved ones shipped home at their own expense. Coffins, caskets, and metal burial cases were supplied by embalming surgeons or local undertakers. Many Union soldiers who were not claimed by their relatives were re-interred in National Cemeteries established after the war. The bodies of Confederate soldiers were often removed to private cemeteries in the South for reburial both during and after the war.

Ice or holding coffins were used as an alternative to embalming as a temporary way to preserve the body for viewing. Ice was placed in compartments in the lid, and a glass window above the face allowed for viewing. The body would then be transferred to a regular coffin for burial.

Temporary Grave Markers

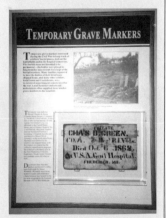

Temporary grave markers were used during the war to keep track of soldiers' burial places, both on the battlefields and in the hospital cemeteries. The burials were not intended to be permanent—the bodies were placed in long trenches and records were kept of the burial locations. Local furniture makers and undertakers often supplied these wooden grave markers to the hospitals.

This marker was made for Private Charles B. Green (Charles Baker Greene), Company A, 7th Rhode Island Infantry. In the fall of 1862 he had become ill with typhus. On October 2, he was admitted to the United States Hotel, part of General Hospital No. 2 in Frederick, Maryland. Greene died on October 6 and was buried in Mount Olivet Cemetery on the south end of town. His body was claimed by his relatives and shipped home, with this marker accompanying the coffin for identification purposes. He is buried in the family plot in the First Hopkinton Cemetery, Hopkinton, Rhode Island. Greene was nineteen years old when he died.

Frederick's Civil War Hospitals

After the battles of South Mountain and Antietam in the fall of 1862, the city of Frederick became a major hospital center. Twenty-seven buildings were taken over for hospital use, two tent hospitals were established, and numerous private homes were used for injured officers. Nearly 10,000 soldiers

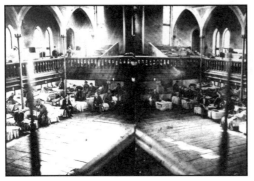

were treated in Frederick in the months after these battles, almost overwhelming the town of 8,000 citizens. Most of the churches, schools, hotels, and other large public buildings were converted into hospitals, and many of the townspeople volunteered their time or resources to aid the wounded soldiers. The Museum building itself was a furniture shop and undertaking establishment during

Top: Interior of the Lutheran Church, 1862, part of General Hospital #4, Frederick. Courtesy of the Evangelical Lutheran Church.

Middle: The Hessian Barracks, c. 1870, General Hospital #1, Frederick. Courtesy of Leib Image Archives.

Bottom: The Jesuit Novitiate, 1854, part of General Hospital #5, Frederick. Courtesy of the City of Frederick.

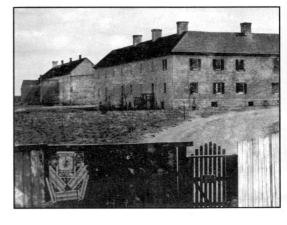

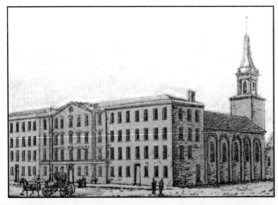

the war and was used as a station to embalm the dead in late 1862.

The Museum has published a book, *One Vast Hospital: The Civil War Hospital Sites in Frederick, Maryland after Antietam*, which details all of these hospitals and includes a patient list for the soldiers treated there in the fall of 1862.

Hospital Ships

In 1862, hospital ships were utilized for transporting the sick and wounded on western rivers, as well as treating them during the journey. The steamers *City of Memphis* and *Louisiana* were the first ships to be chartered for this purpose. Once the usefulness of the hospital ships was realized, many other vessels were put into service, both in the west and along the eastern seaboard. The *Louisiana* was later purchased by the government and renamed the *R.C. Wood*.

The *D.A. January* was refitted for hospital use in 1862 and was considered to be the best-adapted steamer for this purpose. The staterooms were removed to create large and well-ventilated wards, with kitchens, dining rooms, store rooms, and nurses' quarters along the sides. Wash rooms and water closets were placed on each deck, and the entire ship was supplied with hot and cold water.

The hulk of the steamer *Nashville* was also fitted up as a hospital and towed to Milliken's Bend, Louisiana, where it became a stationary hospital. Other ships used on the western rivers included the *Empress, Imperial, Woodford,* and *City of Alton*. On the eastern seaboard, principally along the Virginia Peninsula, ships were used to transport the wounded to the large hospitals in the north. The vessels included the *Daniel Webster, State of Maine, J.K. Barnes, Connecticut,* and *Atlantic*.

The Navy, which had sickbays aboard every ship and land-based Marine Hospitals, also developed a hospital ship, the *Red Rover*. This ship began service in June 1862 on the Mississippi River. Assistant Surgeon George H. Bixby was the surgeon in charge of the *Red Rover*. The hospital staff included religious sisters from the Order of the Holy Cross and a group of African American women who are considered to be the first paid female nurses aboard a Navy vessel.

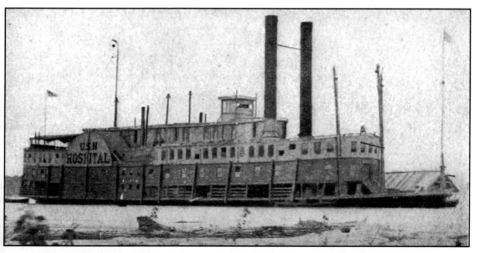

Naval hospital ship the Red Rover. *From* Miller's Photographic History of the Civil War.

Mother Bickerdyke

A window display featuring Mary Ann Ball Bickerdyke was installed at the Museum in November 2001. The exhibit is modeled after an F. O. C. Darley drawing entitled "Midnight on the Battlefield," which is based on an account by a night officer who observed a faint light moving on the deserted battlefield of Fort Donelson, Tennessee, in February 1862. When he sent a guard to investigate, "Mother" Bickerdyke was found checking bodies to make certain none who were still alive were overlooked.

Mother Bickerdyke was one of the most effective, determined, and hardworking nurses who served during the war, and she was beloved by the soldiers she aided. Perhaps the greatest compliment paid to her was, "She looked after me as if I were her son." During her later life, she would remark, "I served in our Civil War from June 9, 1861, to March 20, 1865. I was in nineteen hard-fought battles in the Departments of Ohio, Tennessee, and Cumberland Armies. I did the work of one, and I tried to do it well."

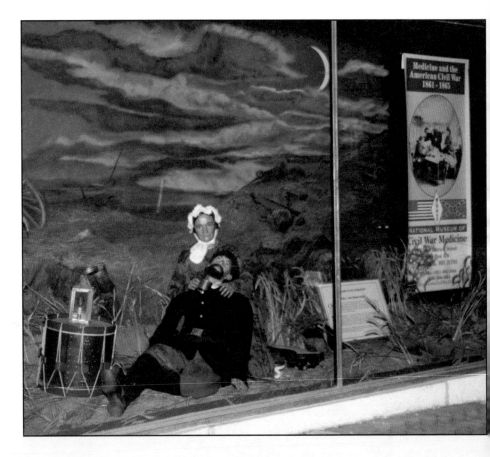

Discovery Stations

Throughout the Museum, there are Discovery Stations with hands-on displays meant to appeal to children. They are aimed for children ranging from 3rd grade to 6th grade. Each station has a similar color scheme and icon of an image of a young boy and girl from the mid-nineteenth century, and each relates to the topic covered in the gallery.

The Discovery Station in the Medical Education gallery asks the visitor to identify human bones through the use of panel doors and four reproduction bones. In the Camp Life gallery, a box contains some typical items a soldier would carry, helping to illustrate the physical hardships endured by the men. In the Medical Evacuation gallery, the hands-on exhibit focuses on the care and feeding of the horses and mules so essential to the armies. In the Final Exhibit gallery, the Discovery Station discusses the roles of children during the war, including drummer boys, powder monkeys, nurses and stretcher-bearers.

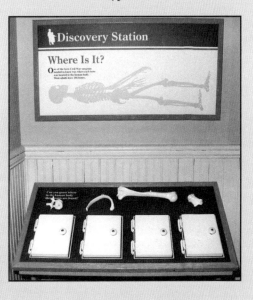

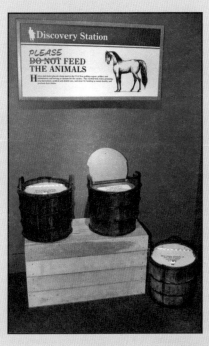

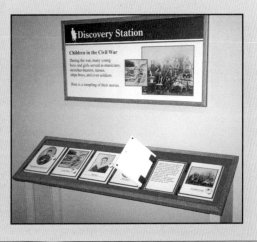

Collections

The Museum houses a world-renowned collection of original artifacts relating to medical care in the Civil War. Most of these historic objects have either been donated to the Museum or are on loan from private collectors and other museums. Many came from the private collection of Gordon E. Dammann, D.D.S. Among the artifacts in the collection are surgical instruments used by Union and Confederate medical staff, various pharmaceutical bottles and containers, medical knapsacks and panniers, stretchers and litters, prosthetic devices, dental tools, various books and documents, a recruiting drum, Union and Confederate surgeons' frock coats, a hospital steward's uniform, a table used for amputations at a field hospital during the battle of Cedar Creek, a Union Army hospital flag, and the only known surviving surgeon's tent from the Civil War.

The Museum has a very narrow scope which directs the acceptance of items into its collection. The mission statement dictates that the Museum can only receive objects specifically related to medical aspects of the Civil War. If an object is deemed acceptable for possible donation, the Board of Directors then votes on whether the item should become part of the permanent collection.

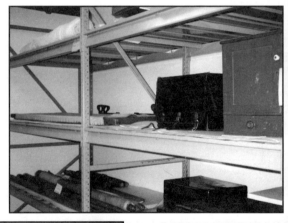

The Museum's collection room houses the artifacts that are not currently on display in a secure, climate-controlled

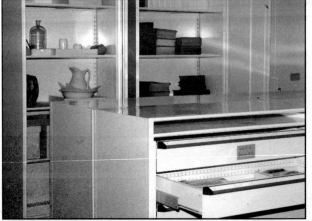

environment. Temperature and humidity levels are kept constant to prevent damage to the objects, and a state-of-the-art storage system ensures their safety. A mix of shelves, drawers, hanging racks and space for large objects was designed to meet the curatorial needs of the Museum.

Wooden Stretcher Bed

Unless a wounded Civil War soldier was capable of making his own way to the surgeon for medical treatment, he would remain on the battlefield until removed by means of a stretcher manned by designated stretcher bearers. During the war, 52,489 litters of various manufactures were purchased and issued to the troops. The most widely used types of stretchers were made of canvas with wooden poles. The Satterlee U. S. Regulation litter was supplied to Union regiments at the beginning of the war. It was soon replaced by the lighter and more compact Halstead litter. Other types of stretchers were made of wood, rope, or cloth. Improvised stretchers of branches and uniform coats were also employed. The wooden stretcher bed on display at the Museum is unusual in that it could be used as a hospital bed as well as a stretcher.

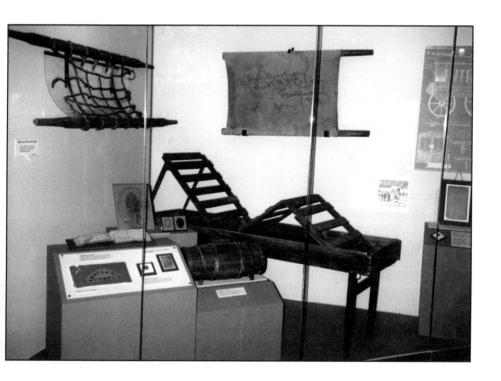

The Squibb Pannier

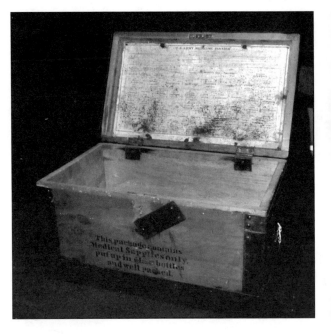

During the first several months of the Civil War, the Union Army used large, heavy chests to carry medical supplies and drugs while on campaign. These cumbersome chests were transported in the wagons of the Army's supply trains and were often inaccessible to surgeons and stewards during an engagement. To remedy this problem, the Army began issuing medicine chests of more compact designs to aid the medical staff on the front lines. One such chest was the Squibb pannier, designed by pharmaceutical manufacturer Edward R. Squibb of Brooklyn, New York. Squibb's panniers were constructed of wood and reinforced with an iron frame, making them sturdy enough to withstand the rigors of march and battle.

A complete Squibb pannier measured 21 inches long, 11½ inches wide, 11⅜ inches deep, and weighed 88 pounds. The pannier was divided into two tiers. Bandages, surgical instruments, and other supplies were stored in the removable upper tier while the lower tier was divided into compartments to accommodate medicines. To make locating a medicine in the pannier easier, each drug container was given a number that corresponded to a numbered compartment in the lower level. A diagram showing the location of the compartments was glued to the inside of the lid for quick reference.

Hospital Knapsacks

Hospital knapsacks were designed for the easy transportation of medicines and bandages into the field. They were the responsibility of the orderly who accompanied the regimental surgeon. There were many types of hospital knapsacks including ones made of wood, leather, and wicker.

The hospital knapsack pictured here is a two-tiered wood and oilcloth pack with leather straps. The top tier is a wooden drawer, which when pulled out gives access to the compartment below. The lower tier is partitioned to accommodate various sized bottles and containers. The bottles are marked "T. Morris Perot & Co.," a Philadelphia firm which supplied medicines to the U. S. Army.

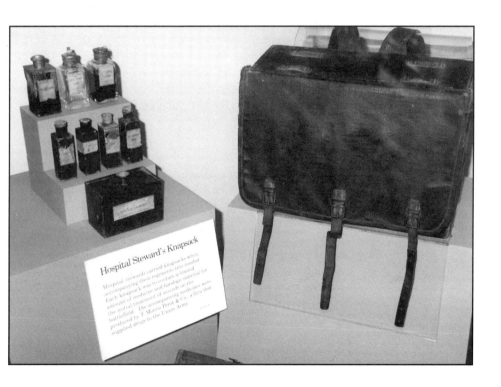

Adhesive Plaster

Adhesive plaster was common among the contents of hospital knapsacks, panniers, and medicine wagons during the Civil War. It had a myriad of uses in the field dressing stations and hospitals. To produce adhesive plaster, resin was added to lead plaster and then spread on one side of thin muslin. The result was a bandage that became adhesive when heated.

Surgeons found adhesive plaster suitable in many applications from the dressing of wounds to the extension and counter-extension of certain fractures. It was frequently used to hold a piece of lint or other bandage material in place or to close the lips of a wound.

Adhesive plaster was produced in rolls and was cut into strips for use. Once cut, the strips were heated to render the plaster adhesive. The necessary heat could come from a variety of sources. Dr. John Hooker Packard wrote, "A very good plan is to have a can of hot water, to the outside of which the back of each strip is applied before it is put on." Warming the strips over a flame from a lamp was another method. Friction from rubbing the strips between one's thumb and forefinger often generated enough warmth for the purpose when other heat sources were unavailable. The strips were then applied as needed.

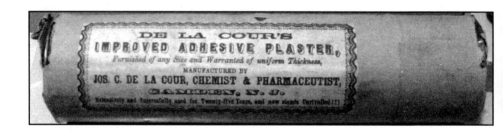

Conservation

From 1999 to 2000, a detailed condition survey of the Museum's collection was carried out. A condition report, treatment proposal and work plan were completed for each object, and each was researched, catalogued, labeled and re-housed in museum-quality storage materials. Artifacts in need of immediate stabilization were treated without delay, while others were given a minimal cleaning and stabilization.

An in-depth study and examination of the paper-based objects in the Museum's collection was done in 2001. The study consisted of identifying the materials, technology and authenticity of over three hundred items and doing a needs-assessment survey which evaluated the condition of the objects and their need for conservation.

In July 1999, four of the Museum's artifacts were selected for the *Save America's Treasures* program by the National Trust for Historic Preservation. The Carty Building that houses the Museum, Surgeon Louis Radzinsky's frock coat, a Confederate pole and rope stretcher, and a Union garrison hospital flag were chosen for this honor. All have undergone conservation.

In February 2000, two of the Museum's artifacts were selected for the *Save Maryland's Treasures* program by the Maryland Commission for Celebration 2000. The items are a Confederate pharmaceutical case and the 1890's freight elevator located in the Museum's historic building. The pharmaceutical case has been conserved.

Hospital Flag

This U.S. garrison hospital flag flew over the hospital at City Point, Virginia. It was brought home after the war by the Surgeon in Charge of the hospital, Robert Loughran of the 80th New York Infantry. Civil War hospital flags are very rare, and this is one of a few left in existence.

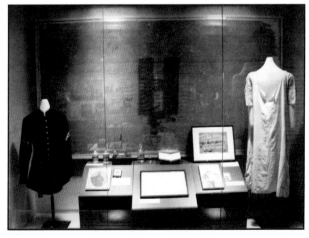

Surgeon John Thomas Parker

John Thomas Parker was born in 1839 in Worcester County, Maryland. He studied medicine at the University of New York and the University of Pennsylvania in Philadelphia. He established his medical practice in Snow Hill, Maryland, then volunteered as a surgeon for the Confederacy during the Civil War. Parker became an assistant surgeon in 1862 and was assigned to Polk Hospital in Atlanta, Georgia. In October 1864, he was assigned to field duty with the 19th Virginia Battalion. Parker was captured on April 14, 1865 and was held in the Old Capitol Prison in Washington, D.C., then transferred to Johnson's Island, Ohio, before his eventual release on June 20, 1865. After his release, he returned to Maryland and to private practice. He practiced medicine until 1912 and passed away in 1917.

A portable Civil War pharmaceutical case that belonged to Dr. Parker is part of the Museum's collection. The case is constructed of wood with brass hardware and contains twenty-nine glass medicine bottles and a set of brass scales. Many of the bottles still hold remnants of their original contents. The pharmaceutical case was conserved in 2001.

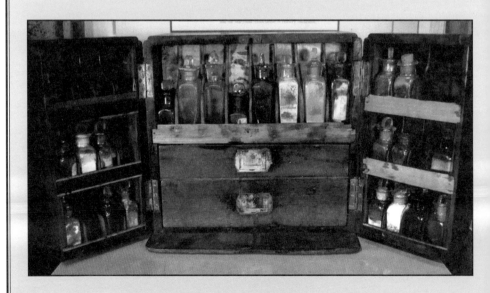

Research Center

The Museum's Research Center is dedicated to advancing the study of Civil War medicine. It contains numerous books, videos, compact discs, DVD's, tapes, microfiche, microfilm and periodicals relating to all aspects of the subject. A special research fund has been created for donations specifically earmarked for buying materials and equipment for the Research Center.

There is also an archival collection of both primary and secondary sources that is organized by subject matter. The archival material has been cataloged and entered into a searchable database which facilitates the retrieval of information. The database includes all of the subjects, people, places and medical procedures mentioned throughout the documents, as well as medical articles from the Civil War-era newspaper *Harper's Weekly*, all of the individuals and hospitals mentioned throughout the Museum exhibits, and all medically-related photographs in the books in the library. The database was designed to make access to the information in the archives easier and more efficient for researchers. The Research Center is open to the public by appointment.

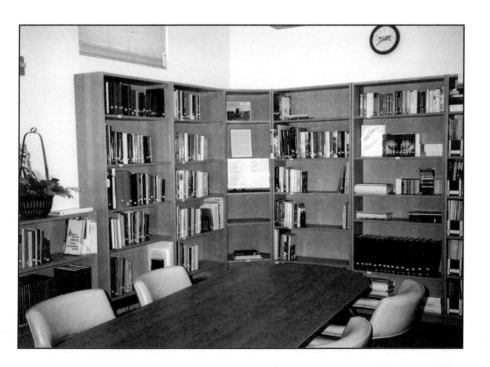

Civil War-Era Medical Terms

Ague:	Chills associated with fever; archaic term for malarial fever.
Apoplexy:	Obsolete term for cerebral stroke, most often due to hemorrhage.
Bilious Fever:	Archaic term for relapsing fever characterized by bilious vomiting and diarrhea.
Blue Pills:	Pills made of elemental mercury mixed with powdered licorice, rose leaves, honey, and sometimes chalk. It was used as a laxative and a cathartic.
Calomel:	Mercurous chloride. Used as a cathartic to induce bowel movements. The use of too much calomel could cause mercury poisoning.
Catarrh:	Inflammation of the mucous membranes with increased flow of mucus.
Consumption:	Tuberculosis; also called phthisis.
Continued Fever:	Obsolete term for fever without the intermittency of malaria; many cases were likely typhoid fever.
Dover's Powder:	A mixture of powder of ipecac and opium; it often included sulphate of potassium and powdered licorice. It was used to treat dysentery, diarrhea and hemorrhage.
Dropsy:	Archaic word for edema; abnormal accumulation of fluid in cells, tissues, or cavities of the body.
Fistula:	Forming an abnormal hollow passage from an abscess or cavity to the skin or an organ.
Intermittent Fever:	A fever that has intervals of complete cessation of symptoms between periods of activity. Often intermittent malarial fever.
Laudanum:	Tincture of opium.
Piles:	Hemorrhoids.
Quinine:	Alkaloid obtained from the South American cinchona tree. Quinine was used to prevent malaria and to lessen the symptoms of malaria sufferers.
Remittent Fever:	A fever where the temperature varies during each 24 hour period but is never normal. Not characteristic of any one disease, but used as a diagnosis in the 19th century.
Resection:	Removal of part of the bone, usually the articular end of one or both bones forming a joint.
Scrofula:	Tuberculosis of the lymphatic glands especially of the neck, characterized by the enlargement and degeneration of the glands.
Trephining:	The drilling or cutting of holes into the skull to relieve pressure on the brain or to remove skull fragments.
Variola:	Smallpox.
Vulnus Sclopeticum:	Gunshot wound.

Educational Programs

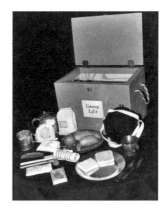

The Museum offers a wide range of educational programs to the public. Docent-guided tours can be scheduled for groups of ten or more. The tours are targeted to the interest level of the group, from grade school through college level and from the casual visitor to the Civil War enthusiast. Tours that focus on special topics such as surgeons or nurses can be arranged.

Various outreach programs are also offered. The Museum maintains a staff of highly-qualified and experienced presenters and lecturers that are available to visit off-site locations. In addition, volunteers set up promotional displays for trade shows, re-enactments, festivals, and special occasions. Other available programs include historical hikes and interpretation of off-site locations relating to Civil War medicine.

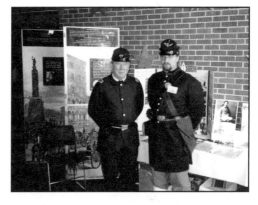

Traveling trunks are available as part of the Museum's educational curriculum. These rental trunks are filled with hands-on projects, reproduction items, photographs, letters, activities, lesson plans and teacher resources. The subjects covered by the trunks include Civil War recruiting and recruitment physicals; camp life (common diseases, nutrition and sanitation); the home-front; battlefield medicine, and triage. In the spring and fall, the Museum holds a series of lectures designed specifically for home-school students. In addition, a guide to the educational resources is available in the Dispensary Store.

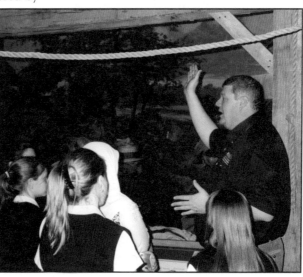

Special Events

The Museum holds a variety of special events throughout the year, including living history programs, lectures, interpretive workshops, art shows, receptions, fundraisers and book signings. Please visit our website, www.civilwarmed.org, for a schedule of upcoming events.

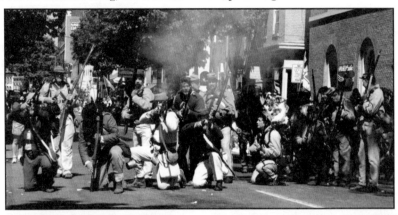

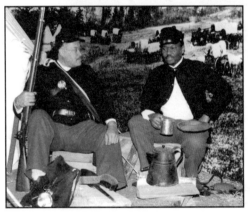

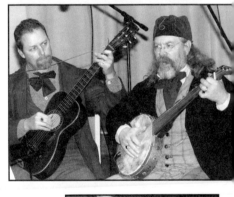

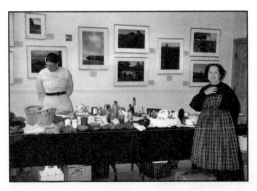

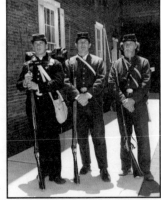

Annual Conference

S ince 1993, the Museum has held an Annual Conference on Civil War Medicine at various locations. The Conference is a scholarly symposium with original papers presented by experts from around the country. It is held over a three-day period and includes the lectures, a field trip to local sites, and social activities. Please visit our website, www.civilwarmed.org, for the latest Conference news.

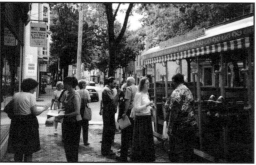

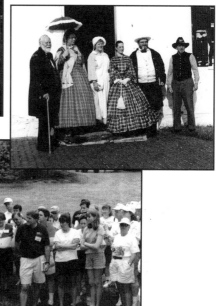

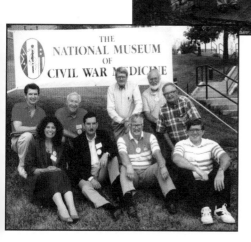

Membership and Support

The Museum has a membership program consisting of nine levels of membership. Benefits for all levels include: individual unlimited free admission for a calendar year, a subscription to the quarterly journal *Surgeon's Call*, a discount on the Annual Conference on Civil War Medicine, and a discount on purchases made on-site in the Dispensary Store.

The levels of membership are: Medical Cadet designed for students, teachers, and home-school parents ($35); Stretcher, individual membership ($40); First Aid Station, two individuals ($50); and Surgeon's Call, membership for descendants of Civil War surgeons ($50). Memberships for four individuals begin at the Ambulance ($75) level and progress to the Surgeon General ($1000) level, with a corresponding increase in benefits.

In September 2003, the Museum started an Endowment Fund which helps provide ongoing support for educational programming and exhibit development. Donations to the Endowment Fund assist the Museum in fulfilling its ongoing mission, educating the public on the story of Civil War medicine.

The Museum is not directly funded by the city, county, state or Federal governments. Any support that is received from these entities is on a grants-only basis. Therefore, the Museum depends on donations from individuals and corporations to maintain its programs and exhibits. Donations are accepted for specific projects and exhibits, as well as for general operating funds. Individuals can donate to the Museum in many ways, including direct contributions, naming the NMCWM as a recipient of retirement plan assets, donation of stocks, and remembering the Museum in a Will. All contributions are tax deductible to the fullest extent allowed by law.

Volunteers

Volunteers are vital to the operation of the National Museum of Civil War Medicine. They serve as greeters working with Museum visitors, act as docents for on-site educational tours, plan and implement the Museum's Annual Conference, assist in cleaning the exhibits, take the traveling displays to outreach activities in the community, serve as hosts at fundraising events, deliver brochures and event calendars, provide clerical support, give lectures for local groups, travel to schools to present educational programs, assist in maintaining the Research Center and assist in research projects, work in the conservation department, do photography, and help in constructing display cabinets.

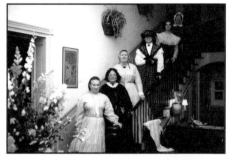

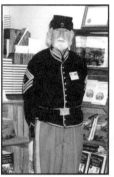
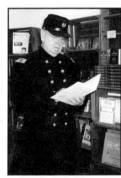

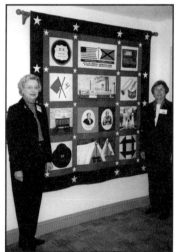

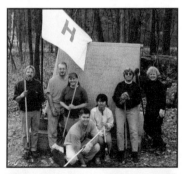

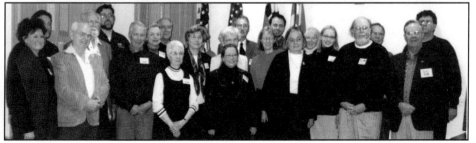

Dispensary Store

The Dispensary Store is an integral part of the Museum experience. Visitors have an opportunity, both before and after their visit, to shop for a variety of items. All of the product carried by the store relates directly to the Museum's educational mission and proceeds support the educational programs and exhibits.

The Dispensary Store carries books, compact discs, videos, periodicals, reproduction Civil War medical items, children's games and toys, clothing and other items with the Museum's logo. Over 250 books are offered, including diaries, journals, and reprints of historic medical manuals. In addition to the on-site store, orders are also taken by mail, phone and on the Museum's secured website, www.civilwarmed.org.

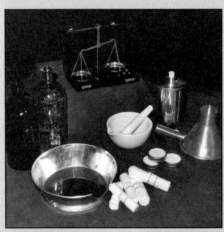

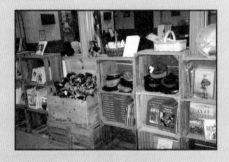

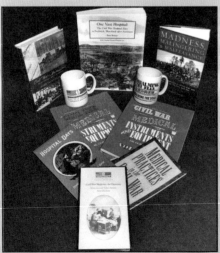

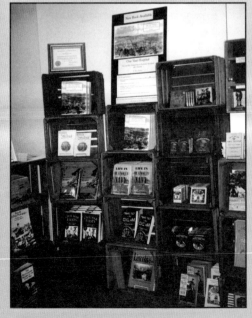

Publications and Videos

I n 2001, *One Vast Hospital: The Civil War Hospital Sites in Frederick, Maryland after Antietam,* was the first book published by the NMCWM Press. It was written by Terry Reimer, the Museum's Director of Research. In 2002, it was awarded a Maryland Historical Trust Heritage Book Award. The book includes a general introduction to Civil War hospitals and staffing, a list of the doctors and stewards at each Frederick hospital, the history of the hospital sites including both a his-

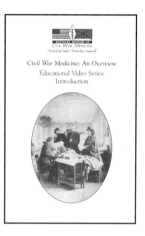

Civil War Medicine: An Overview
Educational Video Series:
Introduction

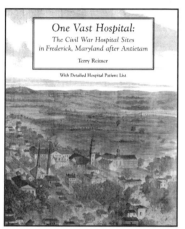

One Vast Hospital:
The Civil War Hospital Sites
in Frederick, Maryland after Antietam

Terry Reimer

With Detailed Hospital Patient List

toric and modern photograph for each, and a complete hospital patient list from after the battles of South Mountain and Antietam. The hospital patient list contains nearly 10,000 individuals and includes their name, rank, regiment, company, complaint, date of admission, date discharged from hospital, and comments. The list is a great source for genealogists and historians.

The NMCWM has produced a video entitled *Civil War Medicine: An Overview, Educational Video Series: Introduction.* The first in a series, it is a general overview of medical practices during the Civil War, where of the nearly 620,000 soldiers who died, two-thirds died not of bullets and bayonets, but of disease. The video explores many aspects of Civil War medicine including: medical education, recruiting, camp sanitation, diet, pharmaceuticals, battlefield medicine, the evacuation of the wounded, amputation and surgery, burial of the dead, the pavilion style hospitals, and the surgeons and nurses. Also available on DVD.

The Museum's award-winning journal, *Surgeon's Call,* is published quarterly and contains news and updates about the Museum, articles on different aspects of Civil War medicine, write-ups of featured artifacts from the collection, upcoming events, volunteer information, and grant updates. It is one of the benefits of all levels of Museum membership.

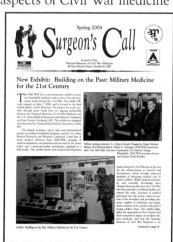

Awards and Partnerships (As of 2003)

Awards

November 17, 1997: Museum receives the first *Joy Reese Derr Award for Outstanding Museum-Community Relations*, presented by the Frederick Historic Sites Consortium

May 1998: Museum commemorated in the United States Congressional Record

July 1999: The Museum's newsletter *Surgeon's Call* wins APEX Award for Publication Excellence

July 1999: Four Museum artifacts selected for the *Save America's Treasures* program by the National Trust for Historic Preservation

February 2000: Two Museum artifacts selected for the *Save Maryland's Treasures* program by the Maryland Commission for Celebration 2000

January 2001: Museum selected by the AAM to be one of eight institutions in the nation to participate as a pilot site for the development of Governance MAP

February 2002: Included in the African American Heritage Sites brochure, Frederick Historic Sites Consortium

March 2002: The Museum's first book, *One Vast Hospital: The Civil War Hospital Sites in Frederick, Maryland after Antietam*, wins a 2002 Maryland Historical Trust Heritage Book Award

September 2002: Placed on the 1862 Antietam Campaign Trail by Maryland Civil War Trails

November 2002: Awarded full accreditation by the American Association of Museums

July 2003: Placed on the Gettysburg Invasion and Retreat Trail by Maryland Civil War Trails

Partnerships

Carroll County Public Schools, Carroll County, Maryland
Frederick County Public Libraries, Frederick, Maryland
Frederick County Public Schools, Frederick County, Maryland
Frederick Historic Sites Consortium, Frederick, Maryland
Greencastle-Antrim School District, Pennsylvania
Hood College, Frederick, Maryland
Mount St. Mary's College and Seminary, Emmitsburg, Maryland
North-South Medical Triangle partnership with Museum of the Confederacy, Richmond, Virginia, and the Exchange Hotel and Civil War Museum in Gordonsville, Virginia
United States Army Medical Research and Materiel Command and Fort Detrick, Frederick, Maryland
University of Wisconsin, Milwaukee

The National Museum of Civil War Medicine Mission Statement

The National Museum of Civil War Medicine is the premiere repository of exhibits and artifacts devoted to the technological and procedural advances made in the medical field between 1861-1865. These changes occurred in the midst of tremendous social and economic upheaval. The Museum is committed to effectively weaving the narrative of suffering soldiers, caregivers, their families and the dramatic and innovative developments in medical treatment. The Museum utilizes its collection to heighten public awareness of the modern medical practices that originated on the battlefields and in the hospitals of this once divided country. Interactive educational programs, exhibits, seminars and lectures provide the knowledge that Civil War medicine connects us not only to our past, but is the scientific and historical link to our present and our future.

Granting Agencies (As of 2003)

The Bank of America Foundation; The City of Frederick; The Community Foundation of Frederick County, Inc; Frederick County; The Frederick County National Bank Donor-Advised Fund; The Frederick Medical Foundation Fund; The Robert E. Gearinger National Museum of Civil War Medicine Endowment Fund; The Institute of Museum and Library Services; The Crosby and William Kemper Foundation, Kansas City, MO; The Kiplinger Foundation, Washington, DC; The MARPAT Foundation, Washington, DC; The Maryland Association of History Museums; The Maryland Historical Trust; Preservation Maryland; The Maryland Humanities Council; The L. J. Skaggs and Mary C. Skaggs Foundation, Oakland, CA; The Small Museum Association, Annapolis, MD; The State of Maryland; The G. Frank Thomas Foundation, Frederick, MD; and the United States Army.

Board of Directors

M. Richard Adams
Edgar G. Archer, Ph.D.
Susan P. Chapin
Gordon E. Dammann, D.D.S.,
Chairman
George B. Delaplaine, Jr., Secretary
Laura E. Estilow, Vice President
Robert E. Gearinger, President
Richard C. Marshall, III
Col. C. James Olson (USA Ret.)
Jonathan F. O'Neal, M.D., Vice
President
John S. Parker (MG/USA Ret.)
Peter H. Plamondon, Jr.
Rev. John W. Schildt
The Honorable Charles H. Smelser
Rev. Armin Weng
Charles R. Zimmerman

Previous Members of Board of
Directors
James F. Doherty
Robert Farmer
F. Terry Hambrecht, M.D., Vice
President
Sam Kirkpatrick, Secretary
O. James Lighthizer
Craig Llewellyn
R. Michael S. Menzies
John E. Olson, President
Charles E. Smith
Cornelius N. Stover. M.D.
Thomas P. Sweeney, M.D., Vice
President
Jack D. Welsh, M.D.
T. Adrian Wheat, M.D., Vice
President
Gretchen Worden, Secretary/
Treasurer

Honorary Board

Edwin C. Bearss
Alfred J. Bollet, M.D.
James O. Breeden, Ph.D.
The Honorable Beverly B. Byron
Shelby Foote
Rev. Roland R. Maust
James M. McPherson, Ph.D.
James I. Robertson, Jr., Ph.D.
Governor William Donald Schaefer

Previous Members of Honorary
Board
Gordon S. Letterman, M.D.
Brig. Gen. Russ Zajtchuk (USA Ret.)

General Counsel
Daniel B. Loftus

Treasurer
Meredith C. Harshman

Executive Directors
George Wunderlich (2002-present)
JaNeen M. Smith (1996-2002)
Burton K. Kummerow (1994-1996)

56

National Museum of Civil War Medicine

48 E. Patrick Street
P.O. Box 470
Frederick, Maryland, 21705

Phone: (301) 695-1864   Dispensary Store phone (301) 695-5225
Fax (301) 695-6823   Dispensary Store fax (301) 360-9782

www.civilwarmed.org
email: museum@civilwarmed.org
Dispensary Store email: store@civilwarmed.org

Open 7 Days a Week
Monday through Saturday 10 a.m. to 5 p.m., Sunday 11 a.m. to 5 p.m.

Closed: New Years Day, Easter, Thanksgiving, Christmas Eve and Christmas Day

Admission is charged. Please visit the website www.civilwarmed.org for admission rates.

Museum Services
  ★ Group tours & outreach programs
  ★ Educational programs
  ★ Special events
  ★ Research Center
  ★ Conference room
  ★ Annual Conference on Civil War Medicine
  ★ Volunteer opportunities
  ★ Memberships available

Location

The NMCWM is located at 48 East Patrick Street in historic downtown Frederick, Maryland, accessible by both I-70 and I-270. A public parking deck is available behind the Museum building. Detailed directions to the Museum are available on the website www.civilwarmed.org.

The National Museum
of Civil War Medicine
48 E. Patrick Street
P.O. Box 470
Frederick, MD 21705
301-695-1864
www.civilwarmed.org

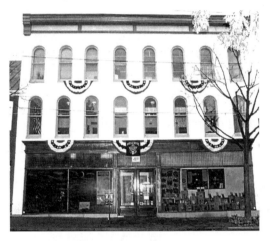

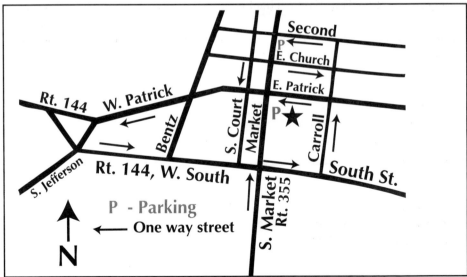

NMCWM Press

The National Museum of Civil War Medicine
is a not-for-profit 501(c)(3) corporation